7 Habits

of

Skinny Woman

by

Subodh Gupta

First Edition February 2013
Copyright ©2013 by Subodh Gupta

ISBN-13: 978-1484008928
ISBN-10: 1484008928

Authored by
Subodh Gupta
+00447966275913
Head office: London (UK)
Email: info@subodhgupta.com
Website: http://www.subodhgupta.com
YouTube: http://www.youtube.com/subodhguptayoga

Publisher Note:
The reader should not regard the recommendation in this
book as substitute advice of a qualified medical
practitioner. The aim of this book is to create awareness
among the masses about healthy food habits. The
information does not endorse any particular brand.

Acknowledgements

I am grateful to my parents and all my teachers who taught me at various stages of my life & shared with me their wisdom.

Content

Introduction:

7 habits of a skinny woman is a story about Olivia's struggle to lose weight.

Since childhood Olivia has felt tired for most of the day and often had low energy level. By the time she was 18 she was already reaching the size 18-20 and her confidence was decreasing day by day.

Over the last 15 years Olivia had tried all kinds of diet plans, magic diet pills, spending money on nutritionists and expensive gym memberships and had even thought of weight loss surgery, such was her desperation to lose weight. This was before she finally met celebrity guru Subodh Gupta, who took her on a journey to lose the weight, gain confidence and become skinny and how Olivia finally attained her dream figure and gained health permanently.

The 7 habits of a skinny woman story is a no-nonsense guide for every smart woman who wants to lose weight, gain health and look fabulous forever.

If you are sick of having extra weight on your body and are desperate to lose it, get ready to become skinny and healthy without drastic measures.

The good thing is that you don't have to starve yourself or stop eating and you don't have to spend your whole life in the gym running on a treadmill but you do need to smarten up.

This book is not about a special diet plan, which in most cases does not work, but rather about the healthy lifestyle of a skinny woman.

Once you adopt a healthy lifestyle you start to become skinny automatically.

This book has 2 parts.

First part of this book contains Olivia's interaction with celebrity guru Subodh Gupta about the habits of skinny woman.

The second part of the book contains tables to record your daily habits so you can note down your improvement. The visual chart will help you to stay motivated when you're having a hard time, when you want to give up.

You will be amazed to see that how easy it is to lose the extra body fat once you follow the Olivia's journey to skinniness.

Healthy habits will lead you to good health and perfect body weight forever.

May all beings be happy & healthy.

Part 1

Skinny Woman Habits

Chapter 1

Practice doesn't make perfect

It is 6am in the morning and the alarm bell is ringing, time for Olivia to get out of bed and start preparing for her work. Thoughts are running through her mind *"I need to take a shower, make breakfast, get ready for work, prepare children's lunch boxes and have a strong coffee to keep me going and I can't see how I can squeeze even 30 minutes of exercising on top of that?"*

She switched off the alarm and lies still in her warm bed. She tries to convince herself that tomorrow she will get up earlier and start her exercise regime.

She doesn't feel she should go to work today and decided to treat herself to a fabulous coffee in the cafe 2 minutes walk from her house. As she was sipping the coffee and enjoying the wonderful sunny day her mind drifted back in time and she started to reflect on her past.

She started feeling that something is missing and that she is not happy with herself. She has put on lots of weight, lost her confidence and often feels tired. She felt lost and helpless and doesn't know what to do.

While flipping the magazine pages something caught her attention. There was a tempting prize to be won by only completing a puzzle and Olivia knew that she was very good at solving puzzles. Without much thought she takes a pen and starts working. When she finishes she feels the excitement spreading in each of her cell. She posts the letter and over the busy weeks forgot about it.

After two months on one fine morning, Olivia's phone starts to ring. She looked at the phone display and sees a private number sign. Generally she never picked up the phone unless she knows the caller so she lets it ring.

The phone rings again and in a spare of a moment Olivia picks it up and she hears a female voice ask "Can I talk to Olivia please? She has won the first prize", "what prize?" Olivia asks. "You have solved the puzzle correctly and you are the winner and you have won a 6 week private consultancy program with celebrity guru Subodh Gupta on *7 habits of a skinny woman and how to gain health forever*".

Olivia couldn't believe her ears. Over the years she had tried all kinds of diets with little or limited success and she really wanted to get rid of the excess body fat she had gained over the years.

Olivia couldn't believe her luck that now she was going to get the opportunity to complete a 6 week program with a celebrity trainer and that it was absolutely free. She felt very happy. This was fabulous news as she was dreaming of having private training for years but delayed it as it was too expensive. Now that she'd got it. She was the happiest woman in the world.

Without any delay Olivia booked her first appointment and reached there half an hour earlier. Waiting at the reception she started thinking that finally she will be able to achieve her dream body.

At exactly 11am, Subodh Gupta arrived wearing a traditional Indian white kurta, Olivia could only think, "Wow! This is it!".

After the introductions, Subodh started the session by asking Olivia, "Do you believe that practice makes perfect?"Olivia had heard this statement before and in excitement said "yes".

Subodh explained that many people mistakenly believe that practice makes perfect but in reality, **practice only makes you permanent.**

This means that "If you keep on practicing in a wrong way you will be permanent in making a mistake instead of getting perfect".

For example, if you are trying to lose weight for years by eating less but still gaining weight and slowly convincing yourself that you can never lose weight. Does this ring a bell? Well it is simply because you are practicing in a wrong way and that's why you are not able to lose weight.

Subodh continued "Skinny woman always ensure that she is practising correctly, hence stays healthy and skinny".

Olivia started thinking, "OMG was I practicing the wrong way to lose weight all my life".

Olivia started thinking that yes it make sense that practice alone doesn't make perfect and *if she keeps on practicing to lose weight in the same way as she did in the past she would stay big.*

As she started thinking about it and analysing it, she got lost in her thought.

"Whether you think you can, or you think you can't — both ways you're right."
— Henry Ford

Chapter 2

Change needed – it's all in our mind

Suddenly Olivia heard "Change needed and it's all in the state of mind".

Subodh explained "It all begins with our belief system in our mind".

He said "Unfortunately many women, after trying hard to lose weight for years but in a wrong way, develop the negative belief system which stops them from becoming skinny".

He added that "Many women have thoughts such as:

-I have tried many years losing weight and I just can't lose weight....

-I am above 50 and my metabolism is slow so I can't lose weight...

-I have fat genes and everyone in my family is overweight so that's why I am too...

-I have thyroid problem and so on... "These negative believes stop them from achieving a "wow" body. If you want to change your body first you need to change your thoughts", said Subodh.

Power of positive thinking:

Subodh suggests that everybody needs to make their own positive affirmation, such as:

"**I am skinny**" and visualize a skinny body in the mind every single day".

"**I am powerful by eating healthy food**".

"**I am a perfect weight**".

"**I am a smaller size**".

Subodh continued: "Imagine your ideal body weight, imagine how you want to look and how you would feel when you achieve that", "Imagine how you might feel when people will compliment you on your ideal body weight".

Subodh said that you will feel good with the affirmation and pleasantly surprised with the positive results.

Olivia believed a little bit in the power of positive thinking and she had heard something about the law of attraction.

Olivia learnt in the past that thought which comes from our belief system effects our blood pressure, respiration, heart rate and physiological process in the body which in turns can affect our weight.

Now Olivia knows that *by changing a belief system she can not only lose weight but also maintain her skinny figure.*

She really wants to fit in her old clothes and she really wants to feel great on top of the world & powerful.

You all have heard **"We are what we eat"** which is correct in addition the following statement is equally true **"We are what we think"**.

If you always picture yourself as big, no matter what you do to become skinny your body will always keep on holding the extra weight", Subodh said.

Olivia realised that if she wants to stay skinny forever it's not only important to change her food but also to change her thoughts, her belief system and her vocabulary.

A skinny woman knows that in order to be slim she must visualise herself slim, always!

Subodh added, "Every woman who is skinny always pictures herself skinny, healthy and keeps **a picture of her role model on the fridge so whenever she is about to open the fridge to eat something she sees her role model** and feels motivated to eat only when needed and only food that is healthy".

Olivia had tried everything, but nothing really worked. She lost some weight but she gained even more each time she did the experiments.

Olivia was using food to make her feel better but it never worked in the long term as after eating food she always felt miserable and guilty.

Subodh asked Olivia to make a point to follow to let go of any negative thoughts and to make a positive affirmation to practice for at least 15 minutes in the morning and 15 min evening.

When Olivia was about to leave, Subodh said, "I haven't finished yet". This is one of the most powerful statements I am going to tell you.

"Every skinny woman on this planet follows that and if you want to be one of them you know what you have to do". "**Nothing great was ever achieved in the history of mankind without discipline and 100% COMMITMENT**"

Olivia learnt that because practice doesn't make perfect and that her old habits are not going to help her to lose weight, she decided to learn new habits. Finally after a long time Olivia started realising that it's time to *change her mind set*.

So she decided to incorporate the positive affirmations into her daily routine and she told herself that no matter what she will commit herself 100 % & practice it every single day.

Olivia noted down in her diary the two habits of a skinny woman.

1st habit – Positive affirmations every day

2nd habit - 100% commitment, no matter what

Chapter 3

Blood sugar balance

Olivia took Subodh's advice seriously and for the whole week practised the mental visualization and positive affirmation process, letting go of her all previous negative thoughts that she can't be skinny. Somehow for the first time in her life she started believing that she can really lose the weight.

Although Olivia still felt low in energy after work (but not in the morning), she was wondering if the positive affirmation could have that much positive impact.

Olivia remembered Subodh's words when he explained that this is a program where you get health forever and you become skinny automatically.

Olivia needed to ask Subodh why she is craving for sugar and feels tired most of the time, why she feels an energy slump in the afternoon and how the skinny women stay energetic all the time.

Before Olivia had even asked Subodh, he told her, "**All those women who became skinny learned the art of balancing their blood sugar level that's why they feel full of energy and don't have sugar craving. Not only did they lose their weight quickly but also kept it off since then**".

Olivia was intrigued that Subodh was able to read her thoughts, how did he came to know what she was thinking and she concentrated her mind on the principles he was explaining to her.

He continued, "To become skinny you need to learn why the majority of people have very low energy level and feel tired, most of the time and how to come out of that way of being".

Olivia felt extremely happy because she was finally going to get answers to her most common problems in her life and felt happy that she can be full of energy now.

Subodh continued, "Cause of low energy is often because blood sugar level is out of control and if she needs to feel full of energy she needs to balance that".

She also needed to figure out what it was that was damaging her eating pattern.

Subodh explained, "**Normally when blood sugar level is low, many people feel tired and hungry and they try to eat chocolate or refined food for fast energy release which cause their blood sugar to rise fast. But since their bodies don't need that much sugar so the body dump the** excess sugar as fat storage and then their blood sugar level falls again which makes them feel tired again, especially with craving for something sweet.

This is how people end up into a circle of tiredness and weight gain".

"*OMG thanks a lot*", Olivia said, "*That is precisely the situation with me*".

Subodh continued, "Symptoms of low sugar level indicates in terms of fatigue, irritation, nervousness, depression, headache and problems related to digestions".

If you want to be skinny and balance your blood sugar level you need to eat food which has low GI.

Olivia felt that today she learned the most important secret of a skinny woman.

"*What is GI Index?*" Olivia asked.

GI index is a measure of how quickly blood sugar levels rise after eating a particular food. Different foods have varying effect on our blood sugar levels.

For example, fresh fruits, vegetables and wholegrain have low GI index but cakes and sweets are high GI index food and they cause havoc in our body.

Mastering your blood sugar level will lead you towards you being full of energy with a skinny body and all you need to do is to ensure you incorporate Low GI index foods in your diet, Subodh explained to Olivia.

Such a simple concept but Olivia was surprised that nobody explained it to her this before as simply as Subodh.

Olivia noted down in her diary that now *she needs to choose food which has a low GI such as oats, lentils, vegetables and fruits.*

She took the decision on cutting down on fast releasing GI foods which resulted in rapid rise in her blood sugar such as: white bread, soft drinks and sweet cereals and replaces them with foods which are of low GI such as, fresh fruits and vegetables.

She will have to give up sugar and carbohydrates and choose wholemeal instead.

Olivia was curious to know if there is any other reason for eating fresh fruits and vegetables. Subodh told her to come to see him next week and put into practice the three habits of a skinny woman she learnt so far.

3rd habit – Incorporate low GI diet

"Nothing will benefit human health and increase chances for survival of life on Earth as much as the evolution to a vegetarian diet".
Albert Einstein

Chapter 4

Fruits and Vegetables

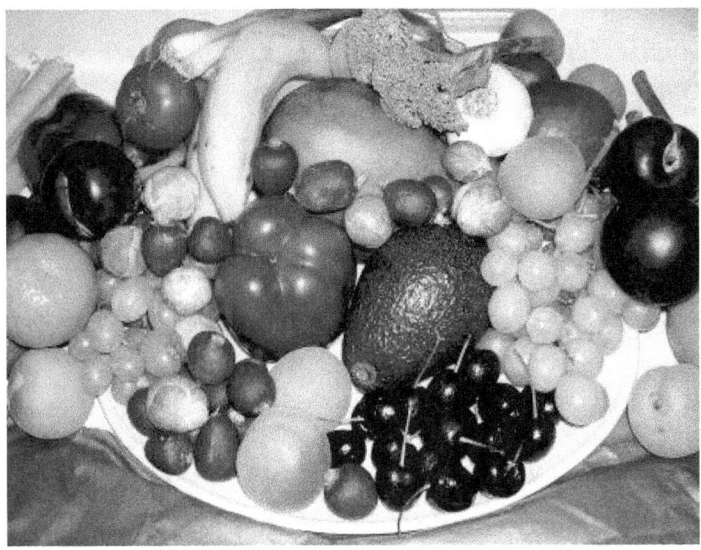

The next week before Subodh could even speak, Olivia asked him with enthusiasm: *"Could you please clarify any health benefits of fruits and vegetable?"*

Subodh smiled his usual smile and pointed Olivia's attention towards a quote on a poster by one of the world's greatest scientist which says:

"Nothing will benefit human health and increase chances for survival of life on Earth as much as the evolution to a vegetarian diet" .***Albert Einstein,***

Olivia had two questions now, *"I understand that you are suggesting to me a vegetarian diet so what should I eat in vegetarian diet?* The second one is *"I have seen many Indian people who are big and even obese and if most Indian's eat healthy food which according to you is a vegetarian diet, why are they obese?"*

Subodh, clarified, "During our six weeks program you need to switch over to the vegetarian diet so you can achieve your skinny body and feel wow. When the program is finished it will be totally up to you which diet you want to follow. You might be surprised which one you choose."

"To answer your second question: **Vegetarian food can also be unhealthy. For example, if you prepare a vegetarian food with lots of oil, it will become fatty and unhealthy similarly in supermarkets lots of fresh vegetable salads are available with the dressing which is often full of fat. So if you eat that salad with lots of fat you are not doing any favour to yourself.**"

Subodh added that "you need to feed your body with lots of fresh fruits and vegetables and **remember to chew your food slowly**".

Olivia looked at the nutritional value of fruits and vegetables for understanding.

Apple 100g average portion can provide 43 kcal and only traces of fat.

Banana 100 g average portion can provide 95 kcal and only 1 g fat.

Orange 160 g average portion can provide 59 kcal and only traces of fat.

Subodh continued "**Fruits and vegetables not only help you to lose weight effectively but also help in warding off heart disease and stroke, control blood pressure and cholesterol and prevent many types of cancer.**

Fruits and vegetables every day are extremely good for the healthy lifestyle.

According to information published on Harvard School of Public Health website titled "Fruits and Vegetable."

"Eating plenty of fruits and vegetables can help you ward off heart disease and stroke, control blood pressure and cholesterol, prevent some types of cancer, avoid a painful intestinal ailment called diverticulitis, and guard against cataract and macular degeneration, two common causes of vision loss."[1]

Similarly according to another article "Scientific studies have shown that people who eat a lot of fruit and vegetables may have a lower risk of getting illnesses, such as heart disease and some cancers. For this reason, health authorities recommend that you eat at least five portions of fruit and vegetables every day." [2]

Fruits and vegetables have many positive effects on our health:

• Their high fibre content helps control blood glucose levels, reduces cholesterol and probably reduces the risk of colon cancer and other cancers.

• They contain antioxidants which may reduce the risk of coronary heart disease.

• They contain essential vitamins and minerals that are vital for good health and disease prevention.

One of the beneficial components of fruits and vegetables is their fibre content. Fibre can calm the irritable bowel and relieve constipation.

Olivia asked, *"How much fruits and vegetable do I need to eat in a day?*

Subodh replied, "The general common advice in terms of eating fruits and vegetables is of five portions a day, however, these five portions should come from a variety of sources every day. If you are interested in losing weight fast, make it to 8 portions a day".

Fruits

To gain the maximum benefit from fruits it is best to eat them fresh. It is better to eat fruits than drinking fruit juices because fruit loses most of its natural fibre in the juicing process.

One portion equal to 80gms:

• Apple, or banana or pear or orange or

• 1/2 avocado or

• 1 large slice of melon or fresh pineapple or

• 3 dried apricots or

• 1 cupful of grapes, cherries or berries

Vegetables

One portion equal to 80gms, which could be a

- 1 cereal bowl of lettuce or

- 1 cereal bowl of salad or

- 3 tablespoons of cooked carrots or peas or sweet corn, etc.

Eating plenty of fruits and vegetables is good for eyes. Vitamin A in carrots helps night vision. **Fruits and vegetables also help in preventing two common aging-**

related eye diseases - cataract and macular degeneration - which afflict millions of people worldwide.

Fruits and vegetables are clearly an important part of a good diet. Everyone can benefit from eating them; however, important point is variety along with quantity.

4th habit – Eat 8 portions of fruits and vegetables everyday

Chapter 5

Metabolism

Olivia said to Subodh, *"I am now convinced with the fact that I need to include daily fresh fruits and vegetables in my diet".*

Olivia told Subodh that she is nearly 38 in October and she heard that after 40 metabolism slows down. She asked Subodh, the health guru, how to increase her metabolism.

Subodh said "To lose weight it is very important for one to have active metabolism and the metabolism can be improved".

(a) First tip to boost metabolism is to **eat regularly** and never miss your b**reakfast** and ensure that in the evening you always eat little because heavy meal eaten especially in the evening always ends up as stored fat in the body.

(b) Never stay hungry for long periods of time because prolong hunger causes body to slow down the metabolism rate.

(c) Spices boost metabolism but that doesn't mean you eat lots of spices and create other troubles in body. Spices should always be used in moderation in the food.

(d) When I advice for **vegetarian food** that is not only because it has low calories but because here is one secret which very few people knows and that is about the process of thermo genesis, production of body heat during metabolism. **Vegetarian has higher rate of metabolism during rest**, which means they burn more calories during rest as body heat.

(e) Lean protein increase the metabolism by up to 10 percent.

(f) Water everyday is a must to speed up metabolism. Fibre speed up metabolism i.e. Fruits is much better than fruit juice.

(g) Exercise increases the metabolism. Women who are skinny always do exercises because they knows that exercise build muscles that increases her metabolism rate because of which she burns more calories even when she is sleeping.

5th habit - Boost metabolism

Chapter 6

Exercise

During her next meeting Subodh asked Olivia about her exercising habit. Olivia felt mortified as *she hated any form of exercises and tried to avoid them as much as possible*. Subodh laughed and laughed at her answer and said that was the common thing many women shared who came to him for help, he explained.

If you want to be skinny you need to move your body **but secret is that you don't have to exercise for hours**. Go for moderate walk or take your dog for a walk or go for swim whatever you loves doing and maintain it.

Workout in the morning is best because in the morning body burn more fat. However, if stuck with any important work in the morning than do your workout whenever you find the time.

Walk for 5 days a week.

"But how should I motivate myself to do exercise if I hate them? asked Olivia.

Exercising with friends improves motivation and specially knowing that your friend is waiting for you outside your house at 6am in the morning make you more motivated. So try to workout with your friends whenever possible.

Subodh asked, "Do you want to feel upbeat about your life or to feel down?"

"Of course I would like to feel better" replied Olivia.

"This is one more reason for you to do a moderate workout because it will lift your mood up and make your immune system stronger so when most of your colleagues suffer from the cold and flu you will stay healthy as your immune system will become stronger by doing a regular workout every day" said the Guru.

Exceptions: There are exceptions when you shouldn't workout, especially when you are ill, injured or having a hangover. When ill or injured your body needs time to heal so rest, however, if having hangover drink lots of water to keep hydrated because a hangover means you are dehydrated. Dehydration means your workout would feel a lot harder so drink lots of water to fight a hangover.

Water

The correct intake of **water** is extremely important for keeping your body free from toxins. In addition it keeps your skin fresh and glowing.

6th habit –Moderate exercise 5 days a week

What else I should do? asked, Olivia sarcastically.

Subodh replied, "You need to give up".

"But why should I give up because you said 100% commitment and I agreed to do that".

Subodh smiled and said:"First focus on what you have learned so far and we will discuss it next week when you come".

As she was leaving, she started wondering *why is he asking me to give up and what has gone wrong.*

"He who does not know food, how can he understand the diseases of man?"

-Hippocrates
the father of medicine (460-357 B.C.)

Chapter 7

Give up

When it was time for her next session, Olivia reached 15 minutes early to meet Subodh as *she was very curious and nervous at the same time*. Olivia loves her daily cappuccino and that is the first thing she does once out of her home for work.

When she met him, she was holding her cappuccino in her hand he smiled and Olivia was beginning to get the idea why he was smiling she thought *if he tries to convince her to give up coffee she is not going to do that.*

Subodh asked Olivia, to remind him what he told her last week,

"*You said that I need to give up*" –Olivia said loudly.

Subodh told Olivia, "I have looked into your diet and what I really want you to do is to give up certain things from your daily meal which you may not like to do but you have to accept this challenge for 6 weeks and later whether you want to continue or not is totally your choice".

Olivia felt a big relief that this it is not about her giving up the daily dose of caffeine. Subodh continued, "If I tell you that there is something which most of us drink, everyday, round the globe and it may result in:

- Gaining weight

- Loss of tooth enamel

- Increased risk of osteoporosis

Last but not the least it may even contain traces of cancer causing elements as well.

Would you drink it?"

Olivia said *"Of course not"*

Subodh continued, "OK Good but have a guess and tell me what many people still drink and that too in huge quantities?"

Olivia was wondering *what could be so dangerous and people still would drink it. She wasn't sure what to say.*

Subodh said "Don' just take my words, but look at what various researches have to say":

As per figure published in Centre for Science in the public interest (CSPI) website about consumption of carbonated soft drink in America "companies annually produce enough soda pop to provide 557, 12-ounce cans, 52.4 gallons-to every man, woman and child".[3] (198.33 litre per person per year, that is almost equal to more than half litre per day per person, 1US gallon = 3.785 litre).

Drinking habit of soft drinks in UK is also not better. "More than 5,560 million litres of carbonated soft drinks are consumed every year in the UK."[4]

He continued, "Let's consider at present UK population is approximately about 60 millions. That means each person in UK drinks about 92.66 litres per year.

It is definitely surprising. It seems that people in America and in the UK drink carbonated soft drinks in place of milk and water".

"Welcome to the world of carbonated drinks",

He explained to Olivia that some of the soft drink products can have up to **210 calories** in each 500 ml bottle along with **53 g of sugar**, flavouring (including caffeine) and phosphoric acid, while other brand products may have less calories and sugar but high amount of **Sweeteners,** Colour, **Preservative** (sodium Benzoate), **Citric acid** along with **Phosphoric acid.**

He explained further that **highly refined sugar is nothing else but chemicals.**

Sugar -> makes you fat, rot teeth, disrupt digestion, and is addictive.

Olivia listened to this new information with horror. She said: "*I have always craved sugar so what can I do?*" Subodh reminded her about the greatness of fruits and told her to eat grapes because Grapes can stop sugar craving.

Subodh continued that many people who crave sugar are low in magnesium, chromium and manganese. -> So

apple, avocados, **almonds** celery, parsley can help in providing magnesium, chromium and manganese.

Subodh told Olivia to do more research and read more about the effects of carbonised drink on human body.

Olivia was surprised to read that *Sugar Sweetened Drink was linked Child Obesity, for example the carbonated soft drinks are the largest single source of calories in American people diet, about seven percent of daily calories intake.*

Not only that these soft drinks are said to have lots of 'empty calories' – they can result in putting on extra weight and don't have much nutritional value.

"A child's odds of becoming obese increase by 60 percent with each additional daily serving of sugar-sweetened drinks".[5] (This was the conclusion of a study from the Department of Medicine at Children's Hospital in Boston and the Harvard School of Public Health).

Carbonated drinks and Human teeth

Olivia knows that people in the UK spent hundreds of pounds for their teeth related issues. She learned that:

"Tooth decay happens when teeth are attacked by acid, and this can happen in two ways. Acid attacks can happen as a result of plaque bacteria acting on the sugars in our diet, or as a direct result of the acids in food dissolving away the enamel on the surfaces of our teeth. As carbonated soft drinks tend to contain

high amounts of both sugars and acids, they're the worst possible combination for dental health."[4]

Olivia was shocked to learn that *while she was enjoying the soft drinks she was giving an "acid bath" to her teeth without being aware of the damage to her teeth.*

She learned that along with soft drinks, sports drinks and energy drinks are also responsible for tooth decay.

Because, most colas contain one or more acids, usually phosphoric and citric acids and sports beverages also contain organic acids which are also known to break down calcium.

The carbonic or phosphoric acid dissolves the calcium out of the enamel and it results into wide scale destruction.

Soft Drinks and Risk of Osteoporosis

As per liquid candy *"Frequent consumption of soft drinks may also increase the risk of osteoporosis — especially in people who drink soft drinks instead of calcium-rich milk..."*.[3]

Another research…

Cancer chemical found in British soft drinks

According to news published on BBC News 24 in Health section *"Traces of a cancer-causing chemical have been found in British soft drinks at eight times the level permitted in drinking water, BBC News has learned"*.[6]

The more she found out the more she wanted to know.

She was reading one research study after another and the terrified truth was revealing in front of her.

One after another research on disastrous results of soft drinks on our body and still how little she thought she is aware of them.

So Olivia decided to give up all kinds of soft drinks because she realised that If she wanted to lose extra weight and gain good health then from this moment onwards she was **not going to drink soft drinks anymore** *for her own good health and she switched to plain still water instead.*

By now Olivia was beginning to understand why Subodh looked so youthful and vital for his age.

She was more and more curious to know what else Subodh had to say about becoming naturally skinny and looking young.

While Olivia had lots on her mind, Subodh was smiling as usual and said:

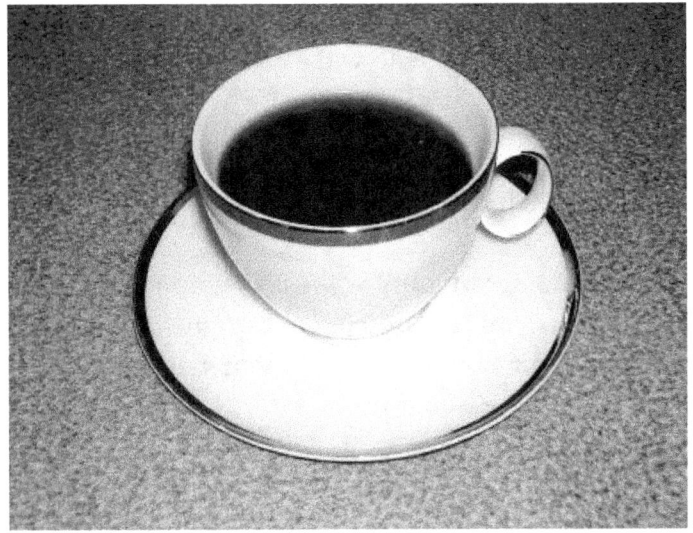

"A Cappuccino, with whole milk 190 g drink can have 65 Kcal with 4 g fat.

A single cup of fresh coffee can give about 80-330 mg of caffeine per cup depending upon type of beans, the way coffee is made and how strong the brew is."

For Olivia drinking coffee was a social and enjoyable activity; a welcome break from work and other activities.

Before Olivia said anything Subodh mentioned that many people believe they need coffee to wake up but in reality they don't need anything to wake up.

Olivia thought again *"Is he reading my mind?"* I was going to tell him exactly what he just said. I need coffee to wake up."

He continued, "**If you can't wake up without coffee, it is because either you are addicted to caffeine or you are not having optimum hours of sleep or you may have over eaten late in the previous night**".

But Olivia interrupted Subodh saying that *"Caffeine makes me feel more alert and awake"*.

Subodh replied, "It can increase your heart rate and pulse. You can feel awake and alert - especially in the morning but if you take higher doses, it may also prevent you from getting deep sleeping".

It is addictive and people tend to rely on it to give them a boost. It can also lead to withdrawal symptoms when stopped taking its consumption.

For example, if you decide to stop taking coffee there is very high possibility that you would experience headaches and drowsiness for couple of days".

Olivia wasn't ready to give up her coffee easily and said that *"most of people can't be wrong because every morning of each day before the office hours coffee houses in London are certainly full"* and *"In Britain about 70% of adults drink coffee and on average each person drinks 3.5 cups of coffee per day*[7].

What I am going to say now about coffee will definitely surprise you Olivia after all those great benefits you might have heard which are propagated by media about coffee:

"Well, **coffee contains caffeine which is addictive and it is one of the world's most widely used drugs which can be the cause of numbers of health problems**. For example:

- It can prevent your body from absorbing vitamins and minerals.

- It can increase the excretion of vitamins and minerals from the body, so you may not get the full benefits of healthy foods.

- It can increase your heart rate and blood pressure.

- It has an impact on the body's energy levels: following the initial energy surge, the levels fall due to the lowering of blood sugar.
- It can cause headaches and insomnia and this is not all".

Coffee & Bad Breath
Have you ever smelt the breath of someone who is a heavy coffee drinker? It certainly doesn't smell nice.

Caffeine & Sleep
If you are having difficulties in sleeping check yourself if you are taking coffee before sleeping.

You would be surprised to know that caffeine could be one of the many reasons for disturbed sleep and of course disturbed sleep is certainly very unhealthy for overall health.

However, the effect of caffeine on sleep varies from person to person.

Caffeine and PMS

According to Jean Carper
Food: Your Miracle Medicine: How Food Can Prevent and Cure over 100 Symptoms and Problems:

"Those consuming at least one cup of a caffeine-containing beverage per day, such as coffee, tea or soft drinks, were more prone to PMS. And the more caffeine they consumed, the more severe their PMS."[8]

Caffeine affects almost entire organ system to the skin. **You need to ask yourself that do you want your skin to get damaged**.

Initially when you give up caffeine, you may experience headache for couple of days but later on it will all be fine.

Olivia was not happy but could see the sense in what Subodh was telling her. She asked him what she should do next.

He told her to initially reduce the number of cups a day or reduce the size of the cups and then begin the day with a glass of lukewarm water with lemon or herbal tea.

Olivia unhappily noted down in her note book that:

*She now onwards has to **minimise her intake of caffeine** and best if she can altogether eliminate it from her food intake and take plain still water instead.*

If she cannot cut down on the number of cups of coffee then, she needs to cut down on the size of cups so she drinks half the quantity.

Fast food

After discussion about coffee Subodh went straight into the topic of fast food. He said to Olivia:

"Becoming skinny or becoming overweight is completely your choice":

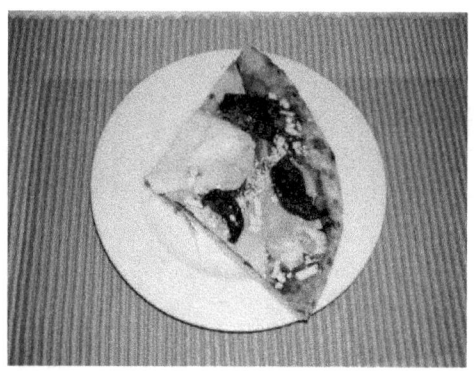

Tomato Mozzarella & Provolone Pizza (V) of 330 g can have **730 Calories**, about **25 g fat** (11.6 g saturated) and 3.6 g of salt (**60 % of salt GDA**)

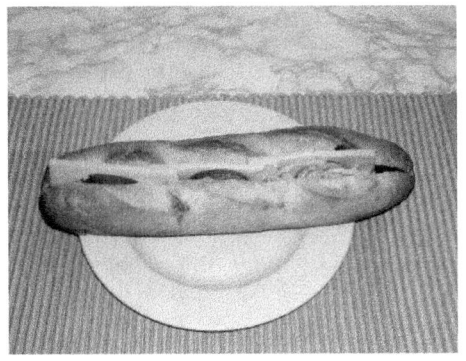

A Ploughman's baguette can provide **603 Kcal**,

23.5 g fat (11.6 g saturated fat) and **3.7 g salt**

Subodh said she has an option to eat what she wants but not the junk food, because **her body doesn't like junk food**.

But *Olivia loves her pizzas and burgers and she doesn't want to get rid of them.* She is started to feel   resentment towards Subodh and she thinks *it's unfair that she can't eat what she wants and by not eating junk food she was making a big sacrifice.*

Subodh said **she needs to think differently that how privileged she is because the healthy food which she can afford is not available to over half of the world population**.

Subodh said that junk food is full of chemicals (which damage our body) and addictives so we eat them more and more". "It is your choice Olivia if you want to damage your body"- he said without any sympathy.

Olivia now has to make a choice, a choice between a diet without any junk but which gives her a wow skinny body or a junk diet with lots of extra fat on her legs, arms and tummy.

Olivia still is not happy, so Subodh continued...

"Eating at Fast-food Restaurants More than Twice per Week is Associated with More Weight Gain and Insulin Resistance in Otherwise Healthy Young Adults" [9]

This extra weight puts you at risk for developing many diseases, especially heart disease, stroke, diabetes, and cancer, etc. So fast food is helping you to gain weight and put you in danger of losing health.

He further explains to Olivia that **most fast food is very dense in calories and a diet high in fast foods will decrease your hope of becoming skinny and you may end up gaining weight.**

He said, most of the food does not have any nutritional value at fast food joints and the menus still tend to include foods high in fat, sugar and calories and low in fibre and nutrients. For example, a Tomato Mozzarella & Provolone Pizza (V) of 330 g can have **730 Calories**, about **25 g fats** which is very high and almost half of it saturated.

He added indulging in fast food brings extra weight along with it. By the end of the day the choice is always yours.

If you are looking forward to lose weight, you need to **Avoid Fast Food**.

Olivia learned that she needs to love the food that her body needs and wants. She needs to love the food which keeps her slim and healthy and she needs to give up fast food.

Next week when she reached Subodh's office she finds a new poster on the wall and she was sure it wasn't there last time when she came to visit him.

"You put a baby in a crib with an apple and a rabbit. If it eat the rabbit and plays with the apple, I will buy you a new car."

-Harvey Diamond

She started thinking *"Is this poster for me. What does it mean?"-*

Meat

Subodh said that today we will talk about meat.

"Is there something wrong with meat?" She felt that her temper was rising. She was born into a family that ate meat every day and she has been eating meat every single day since her childhood.

Olivia said with anger *"Mr Gupta I know you are vegetarian but if I told you that vegetarian food is unhealthy would you accept it?"*

The health Guru replied "No",

"So why should I accept your point which you are going to make about meat?."

She continued *"Every single research you are going to put in support of vegetarian food , I can also put the same number of research report in favour of meat and I don't want to leave that aspect of my diet and I don't want you to explain to me that meat is not good for me"*.

Subodh smile as usual and said, "I am not asking you to leave meat, you can continue your meat diet once you become skinny, until then you need to take up a challenge and give up meat for the six weeks.

Olivia felt better thinking that six week is not that long and she took up the challenge. She could continue with her meat diet once she finished with the course, however she was bit curious and *asked Subodh if he could please explain why he was asking her to avoid meat for six weeks.*

He replied "**Most of animal foods are higher in fat content** than most plant foods, particularly saturated fats. For example fat content in Lamb (breast, untrimmed, roasted) of 90 g average portion is about 27 g fat which is too high. Similarly about 100gms of meatloaf contains 11g of fat but *for a healthy weight loss diet,* I would recommend that one should go for food which has fat content less than 5 %."

"So if you are eating meat regularly, there is very high possibility that you would gain weight apart from developing issues related to digestion".

In fact as per study published on *Magazine* Physician committee for responsible medicine under titled "*Meat-Eaters Gain Weight*" "A new study confirms that meat-eating encourages weight gain. **Researchers from the American Cancer Society studied 79,236 young and middle-aged men and women,** measuring their diets in 1982 and again in 1992. Those who ate more than three servings of meat per week were much more likely to gain weight as the years went by, compared to those who tended to avoid meat". [10]

Another research by the *Vegetarian & Vegan Foundation (VVF)* shows that "meat and dairy are at the core of the world's expanding obesity epidemic..." "*The American* Cancer Society followed 75,000 people over a decade and found that one food was most associated with weight gain – **meat**".[11]

Meat is largely deficient in vitamins except for the b-complex.

"Meat is very high in protein but have no fibre (which should be part of healthy diet). "For weight loss or to maintain the healthy weight, one needs fibre rich food with less than 5 % fat content while meat contains about 10 to 20% fat without any fibre. At least our Weight Loss program and meat cannot go together".

But Olivia interrupted Subodh, *"Isn't it true that vegetarian don't get enough protein?"*

"That is another myth" replied Subodh. If your statement is true than in a country like India where the majority of populations are vegetarian majority should suffer from Protein deficiency isn't it is? Well that is not the case. On the contrary too much protein especially animal protein has potential to damage our kidneys. Vegetable food such as whole grains, lentils and soya products provide sufficient protein for our body.

Subodh said, "The lack of awareness is natural if you were eating what your parents thought is healthy for you and you were brought up thinking that having a beef burger or ham sandwich is a natural way of living.

Now as an adult you have the choice to decide what is healthy for you.

Making the right decision would certainly help you to lose weight and stay healthy forever."

Olivia's anger started subsides as her quick thinking brain begins to connect the information, though she may not agree with him 100% but decided to leave meat for 6 weeks program.

Many things made sense to her already and she would be stupid not to try this 6 week program which she won anyway.

Nothing to lose and may be something to gain. There were things she wasn't agreeing to or convinced but suddenly she saw Subodh putting short quotation written on a white paper from her favourite Paul McCartney in front of her which says,"

"We stopped eating meat many years ago. During the course of a Sunday lunch, we happened to look out of the kitchen window at our young lambs playing happily in the fields. Glancing down at our plates, we suddenly realised we were eating the leg of an animal who had until recently been playing in a field herself. We looked at each other and said "Wait a minute, we love these sheep - they're such gentle creatures. So why are we eating them?" It was the last time we ever did."

- Paul and Linda McCartney

"Wow, it seems you know everything." she looked at Subodh.

He said laughingly "Not everything, my English grammar is very weak".

Subodh then gave her another statement to read by one of the world's most renowned M.D. which says,

"The beef industry has contributed to more American deaths than all the wars of this century, all natural disasters, and all automobile accidents combined. If beef is your idea of 'real food for real people,' you'd better live real close to a real good hospital."

--Neal D. Barnard, M.D., President Physicians Committee for Responsible Medicine

"OK, Ok, you won. This is completely new to me but I will keep my mind open. I am ready to give up meat for the duration of your program".

"That's only what I am asking you to do, 100% commitment at least till the program".

The next discussion is focussed on alcohol and its impact on health.

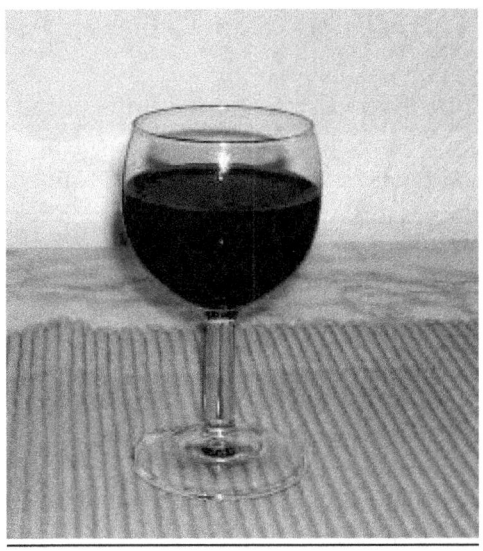

If you drink wine everyday even under the safe limit, still you would end up putting on at least 26 pounds of extra weight each year.

Alcohol

Many times I came across people who ask me "Mr Gupta, I have been eating healthily but still I can't shed those extra pounds". My answer always starts with the same question: "How much alcohol do you drink?"

So Olivia, *"Oh, I don't drink a lot"-Olivia face turned pink. "Maybe 5-6 glasses of wine each week."*

"Alcohol = Lots of empty calories"- the Guru said.

"For example; if you drink about 3 units of red wine a day (Safe limit for woman as advised by department of health UK- Not more than two to three units a day) that means about 255 empty k calories a day in your body, which means 7650 k calories each month.

That means you can easily put on 2.18 pounds each month which may result in 26.23 pounds of extra body weight each year just by drinking red wine everyday even under safe limit as per the guideline by UK govt."

Yes you have read it correctly "If you drink wine everyday even under the safe limit, still you would end up putting on at least 26 pounds of extra weight each year."

The worst effect alcohol has on our weight is that it removes our inhibitions, so we eat and drink much more than we need or plan to.

- Alcohol helps fat to be absorbed effectively.

- Alcohol, especially white wine and champagne enhances your appetite. *So if you drink it before the meal, surely you would end up eating more and hence the extra weight.*

- *Alcohol tends to dehydrate you and dehydration can slow your metabolism, preventing weight loss.*

Another point to consider is that alcohol does not affect everyone in the same way. **Women and older people will generally be at greater risk of these effects even at lower levels of consumption.**

But Olivia said that research studies show *there are health benefits of alcohol consumption.*

"Yes you are right" said Subodh, "but only when you take it in moderation. However, the issue is that alcohol is very addictive and most of the time people end up in excessive drinking because the mind loses its control and when the mind loses control, you can't achieve anything.

Excessive drinking of alcohol has also been linked with some type of cancers, malnutrition because of changes in digestion and metabolism, muscle cramp, depression and osteoporosis, etc."

How many units?

UK Government department of health advises: Men should not regularly drink more than three to four units a day: 3–4/day; and women not more than two to three: 2–3/day; Of course, in some situations like pregnancy, avoid drinking alcohol completely.

*My recommendation for alcohol intake is different than the UK Heath Department advice. Make sure you **never drink more than once a week and you do not exceed more than 2 units.***

I know Olivia what you might be thinking now: "If I drink only 2 units I am not going to enjoy it." "I can assure you that you will have the same enjoyment with 2 units which you experience normally after 8 to 10 units because your body would have been detoxified by following healthy habits."

"However, during the first six weeks you need to say a big no to alcohol", later you may drink it responsibly" –Gupta said.

Chocolate

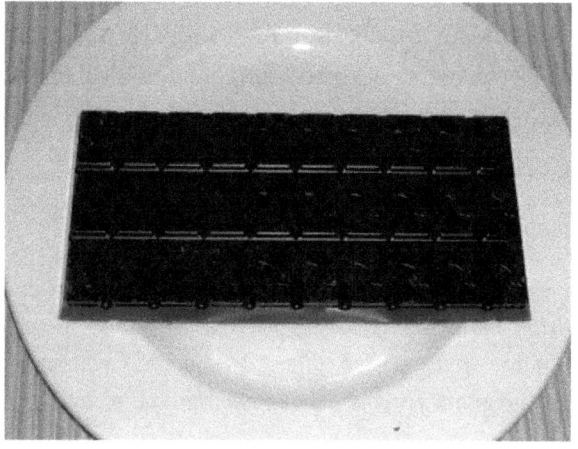

A smooth milk chocolate of 200g can provide **1082 Kcal, 112 g sugar** and **64 g Fat (38 g Saturated Fat)**

Subodh told Olivia that their journey towards healthy weight loss is almost over. He assured her that she was a great student who questioned everything but at the same time kept her mind open to new learning and challenges.

"Now we will talk about Chocolate cakes and crisps"- Gupta said.

"Olivia you need to understand one fact that **you are more special than the cake, crisp and chocolate** and you should eat food which keeps your body healthy and skinny."

To everyone who is interested in losing weight, one thing needs to be clear - you need to get rid of products like fast food, chocolate and crisps especially when you are trying to lose weight.

The chocolate has lots of calories is small portion because it is a dense calorie food. In fact chocolate / crisps not only contain many calories but also unhealthy fat and lots of sugar.

A potato crisp some of us may think that are healthy potatoes cooked in sunflower oil and is a perfect snack.

However, the reality is most crisps consist of *trans fat* and *masses of chemicals* and they are not natural as you may think. Many crisps are just mashed potato mix and a cocktail of additives.

"Olivia I would say in brief that **avoid Chocolate / Crisps/Cakes** and if you cannot avoid them then please eat them only once in a while but certainly not as a regular snack."

The frustration was visible on Olivia's face."You have said no to almost everything I used to eat so could you please tell me what I could eat.

"The list will be long-Olivia", said Subodh smilingly, *"Fruits, vegetables, wholemeal food, seeds, soya products, etc."*

Subodh didn't feel offended by Olivia's attitude because he knew that was supposed to happen. It happens with every client he had and he was used to it.

After a week of initial difficult time, Olivia is finding very easy not to indulge in fast food. She learned a technique that when the craving was coming for certain unhealthy food she associated that food with hate/dislike. She remembers Subodh's words – "**Simply associates pain or hate with any food to avoid craving for it**".

Olivia remembered Subodh's explanation, he said to Olivia "think for a moment that you are about to eat your delicious dish and somebody might cough on that dish or sneeze on that dish, within a moment you will have aversion for that dish even though you love that dish" so by associating dislike and hate you can stop craving that food.

"I have one last question for you. How can millions of people worldwide eat meat products, fast food, chocolate & crisps, etc. and be wrong?"

Subodh replied, "Great Olivia that you asked me this question. **Marketing of unhealthy products is so powerful that majority of people choose to buy those foods and just assume that majority cannot be wrong**; I eat and drink what everybody else does and everybody cannot be wrong."

"Think about it Olivia if this kind of eating habit is healthy then why obesity is increasing like never before in the western nations? Why so many people are falling ill and dying even though the medicine world is so advanced? Have an open mind and think for yourself".

"You might be thinking, well there can be many other factors as well responsible for all these diseases. Yes you are right. There are combinations of factors which are responsible for ill health but the point to emphasise here is - **our food is the most important aspect in all these factors because our body is made up of food we eat**.

If we take out unhealthy food habits and replace them with healthy one we will lose weight naturally and gain health forever without much effort.

The only way to live a healthy life and have perfect body weight is to have healthy eating and drinking habits."

Healthy Food Habits = Good Health + Perfect Body Weight *Forever*

Olivia realised that *she needs to give up her unhealthy habits and change them for the better one.*

Olivia realised that *most of the things she eats was because of how the food made her feel.*

Finally Olivia told her mind that *she wants to be skinny more than she wants to eat the cake.*

Olivia realised that eating cake or chocolate will may make her feel good, momentarily, but *by avoiding cake or chocolate and becoming skinny and healthy will make her feel good for ever.*

So she started making notes of her past habits and figure out which one may not be working and finally made the resolution that *she needed to give them up for a period of at least six weeks.*

7th habit: Skinny woman generally avoids soft drinks, coffee, cakes, sweet, chocolate, crisps, high fat meat products and drink alcohol responsibly.

In the end Subodh suggested Olivia to follow these 7 habits of a skinny woman for 6 weeks and write to him, her success story at: info@subodhgupta.com. He also promises that her success story will be published on Obesity Campaign UK portal so she can be a role model for others.

<u>Note:</u>

You would feel benefit

only

when you incorporate 7 habits
into your life.

Part 2

Recording Improvement

Wellness Monitor

Before beginning 7 habits plan, please take couple of minutes to fill in the following wellness monitor.

	Wellness Monitor	
S.N.	Indicators	Before starting
1	Blood Pressure (High)	
	(Low)	
2	Hours of sleep per day (average over a week)	
3	Quality of sleep (1 to 10) (1 lowest and 10 the best, average for the week)	
4	Body Weight Waist Measurement	
5	Overall energy level (1 to 5) (1 lowest and 5 highest)	

Daily Habits Record

Week 1

Starting Date ....

S.N.	7 Habits	Sun	Mon	Tue	Wed	Thu	Fri	Sat
1	Positive affirm							
2	Low GI Food							
3	Fruits & Vegetables							
4	Metabolism							
5	Exercise							
6	Give up junk food							
7	100% commitment							

Daily Habits Record

Week 2

S.N.	7 Habits	Sun	Mon	Tue	Wed	Thu	Fri	Sat
1	Positive affirm							
2	Low GI Food							
3	Fruits & Vegetables							
4	Metabolism							
5	Exercise							
6	Give up junk food							
7	100% commitment							

Daily Habit Record

Week 3

S.N.	7 Habits	Sun	Mon	Tue	Wed	Thu	Fri	Sat
2	Low GI Food							
3	Fruits & Vegetables							
4	Metabolism							
5	Exercise							
6	Give up junk food							
7	100% commitment							

Daily Habits Record

Week 4

S.N.	7 Habits	Sun	Mon	Tue	Wed	Thu	Fri	Sat
1	Positive affirm							
2	Low GI Food							
3	Fruits & Vegetables							
4	Metabolism							
5	Exercise							
6	Give up junk food							
7	100% commitment							

Daily Habits Record

Week 5

S.N.	7 Habits	Sun	Mon	Tue	Wed	Thu	Fri	Sat
1	Positive affirm							
2	Low GI Food							
3	Fruits & Vegetables							
4	Metabolism							
5	Exercise							
6	Give up junk food							
7	100% commitment							

Daily Habits Record

Week 6

S.N.	7 Habits	Sun	Mon	Tue	Wed	Thu	Fri	Sat
1	Positive affirm							
2	Low GI Food							
3	Fruits & Vegetables							
4	Metabolism							
5	Exercise							
6	Give up junk food							
7	100% commitment							

Wellness Monitor

After completing your 6 weeks 7 habits plan, please take couple of minutes to fill in the following wellness monitor and compare that how you have improved on the following parameters.

	Wellness Monitor	
S.N.	Indicators	After 6 weeks
1	Blood Pressure (High)	
	(Low)	
2	Hours of sleep per day (average over a week)	
3	Quality of sleep (1 to 10) (1 lowest and 10 the best, average for the week)	
4	Body Weight Waist measurement	
5	Overall energy level (1 to 5) (1 lowest and 5 highest)	

Reference:

(1) Harvard School of Public Health "Fruit and Vegetables"
<online>
http://www.hsph.harvard.edu/nutritionsource/fruits.html

(2) Stinton M, BBC Health "Fruits and Vegetables"<online>
http://www.bbc.co.uk/health/healthy_living/nutrition/basics
_fruitveg1.shtml

(3) Centre for Science in public interest (CSPI), "Liquid Candy:
How soft drinks are harming America's health"<online>
http://www.cspinet.org/liquidcandy/

(4) Greenhalgh, Alyson, "Carbonated soft drinks" <online>
http://www.bbc.co.uk/health/healthy_living/nutrition/drinks
_soft2.shtml

(5)United States National Institute of Diabetes and Digestive and
Kidney Diseases (NIDDK), "Study Links Soft Drink
Consumption to Childhood Obesity"<online>
http://win.niddk.nih.gov/notes/winnotesfall01/studylinkssoft.
htm

(6)BBC News 24 "Health: Cancer chemical found in drinks" 1st
March 2006 <online>
http://news.bbc.co.uk/1/hi/health/4763528.stm

(7) Leeds Student Medical Practice" Health Advice: Caffeine"
<online>
http://www.leeds.ac.uk/lsmp/healthadvice/caffeine/caffeine.
htm

(8)New Target, "The health effects of drinking soda - quotes
from the experts" January 08, 2005 <online>
http://www.newstarget.com/004416.html

(9) US department of health and human service, National
Institute of health "Eating at Fast-food Restaurants More than
Twice per Week is Associated with More Weight Gain and

Insulin Resistance in Otherwise Healthy Young Adults" 30th
December 2004 <online>
http://www.nih.gov/news/pr/dec2004/nhlbi-30.htm

(10) The Physicians Committee for Responsible Medicine
"Magazine, Obesity: Meat Eaters Gain Weight "autumn 1997
volume 6 number 4, <online>
http://www.pcrm.org/magazine/GM97Autumn/GM97Autum
n12.html

(11) Vegetarian & Vegan Foundation "Write to Fight Flab:
Government Urged to Face-Up to Real Cause of Obesity"
<online>
http://www.vegetarian.org.uk/campaigns/globesity/letters.ht
ml

Our other published books:

Gentle Yoga for 50 Plus

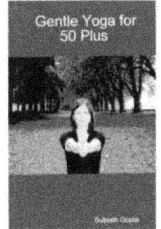

"A perfect <u>gift</u> of health <u>for your parents</u>"

The only book on Gentle Yoga for people in the age group of 50 plus. The exercises explained in this book are also beneficial if suffering from **arthritis** or **rheumatism**.

ISBN 978-1-84799-149-2

Paperback/ £5.95/ 68 pages | Kindle edition £2.98 only

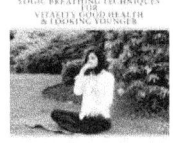

Yogic Breathing Techniques for Vitality Good Health & Looking Younger

The only book on Yogic breathing techniques **for enhancing vitality and looking younger** with clearly illustrated photographs.

This book is ideal for anybody who leads a hectic life style. The simple breathing techniques described in this book will help you to reduce your stress level and improve health.

You will feel the difference by practicing 10 min every day.

http://www.amazon.co.uk/Breathing-Techniques-Vitality-Looking-ebook/dp/B009KIWLIC

Kindle edition @ £2.98 only | Paperback edition £6.95 only

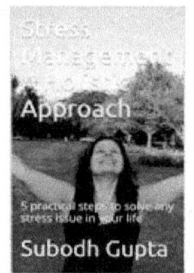

Stress Management a Holistic Approach

5 Steps plan to manage any Stress issue in your life

Many illnesses such as diabetes, migraine, asthma, ulcer and even cancer arise because of excessive Stress over the period of time.

You may have any kind of problem or issue in your life, once you follow the 5 steps described in this book you are on your way to Stress free life. **If there is a problem then there has to be a solution and this book is all about solution.**

ISBN 978-0-9556882-1-8 | Page 80 / Paper Back / £4.95

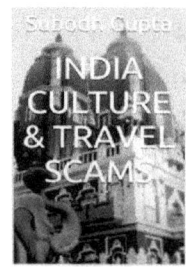

India Culture and Travel scams

"The only book on travel scams targeted at western tourists in India"

This book offers illuminating insights into the Indian culture and society and will help you to turn your India visit into a memorable and enriching experience.

This book will help you to feel more confident in unfamiliar situations.

Content in this book includes Indian social customs, their perception about Western women, religion, travel scams targeted at Western tourists, etc.

http://www.amazon.co.uk/India-Culture-Travel-Scams-ebook/dp/B00DX5DFC4 **Kindle edition @ £2.99 only**

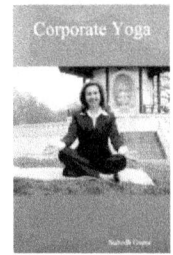

Corporate Yoga

"The Only Book on Corporate Yoga"

This simplified book of corporate yoga has been written considering the need of people working in the corporate sector.

This book will help in relieving pain from lower back, neck, fingers and forearms. It will also help in making eye muscles stronger, releasing stress and keeping the blood pressure normal.

ISBN 978-0-9556882-2-5
Page 96 / Soft Cover / £19.95

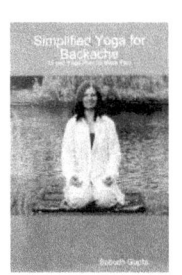

Simplified yoga for backache

Yoga for Back Pain Simplified.

This book is a **carefully** designed practical guide for preventing and managing back pain.

Majority of back pain are caused by muscular insufficiency and lack of flexibility. Yoga poses described in this book will strengthen your back muscles and greatly improve your flexibility. **Simple yoga poses described in this book can be practiced by everybody, whether young or old, beginner or advanced.**

Kindle edition £2.98 only | Paperback edition £4.95 only

http://www.amazon.co.uk/Simplified-Yoga-for-Backache-ebook/dp/B00DV1OO4S

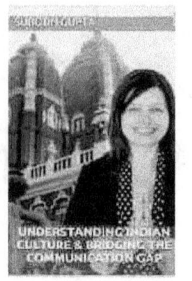
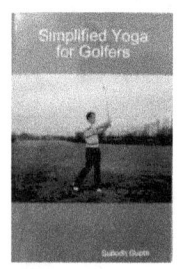

Wellness workshops at workplace in London

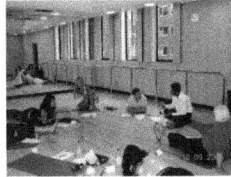 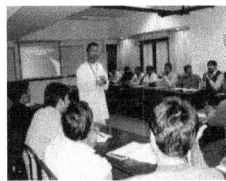 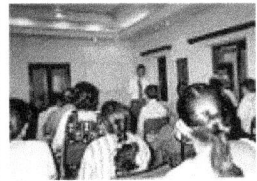

We provide following wellness workshops and classes for corporate organizations in London.

(1)Yoga classes

(2) Half day workshop on Work Life Balance

(3)Half day workshop on Stress Management

(4)Half day workshop on Weight Loss and Nutrition

**For details please contact: Barbara Tomasik
44(0)7966275913 (London) or barbara@subodhgupta.com**

or

Please visit our website: http://www.subodhgupta.com

http://www.celebrity-personal-trainer.co.uk

Connect with us at:

https://twitter.com/celebrityyoga

http://www.youtube.com/user/subodhguptayoga

https://www.facebook.com/pages/Motivation/284494454921356